The Business of Dental Hygiene

How to Create a Hygiene Driven Practice

Wendy Briggs, RDH

Publisher: Hygiene Diamonds www.HygieneDiamonds.com

ISBN-13: 978-0692723661
ISBN-10: 0692723668

DEDICATION

This book is dedicated to my better half, Travis Briggs. This journey would not have been possible without your unconditional support and encouragement. You made it possible for me to follow my dreams.

To my children, Kati and Rob, Keegan, Tate and Quin. You are my everything and inspire me in all I do.

CONTENTS

ACKNOWLEDGMENTS

Dr. Wally Andelin, who gave a young girl a chance to work in dentistry and introduced me to the profession I love. Dr. Moody and Nielsen, who gave me a wonderful dental home to develop my skills. I still miss working with them every day! Dr. Ross Cheesman who first suggested that we could help others by sharing our knowledge consulting with dental professionals. Dr. John Meis, a mentor and friend from whom I have learned so much. Dr. Tom Orent, Tony Gedge, Dr. Woody Oakes, Jack Abrams, Ed O'Keefe, Dr. Dave and Jill Sisson, Dr. Phil and Caron Stein and all the gurus who helped introduce me to the dental community. Dr. Ken Molen for understanding my vision and helping educate a new generation of hygienists to serve patients at the highest level. The incredible team at Henry Schein Dental, Tim Sullivan, John Chatham, Eric Nuss and the incredible BCS team for all your support.

I couldn't survive without the support and work of Bert Triche, Kristie Kapp, Laurie Kimball, Karie Garman, Holly Mitchell, Heather Driscoll, Cathy Ariana, Brad May, Sydnee Merrill, Karen Skorey, Kati Smith, and Angie Baker and the incredible team who are busy making magic happen behind the scenes.

My parents, John and Cathy Atherton, who encouraged me to work hard and taught me resourcefulness and creativity.

Last to my friend Darcy Juarez for always pushing me to accomplish big things.

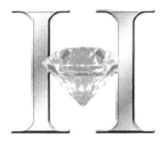

CHAPTER 1

The Business of Dental Hygiene

<u>This book is not written</u> for hygienists. While there may be some hygienists who find great value in what you are about to find here, you must know that this book is written for the dentist who is looking to grow their practice, the dentist who has the desire and ability to change the way their practice treats patients.

This book is written for the practice owner who wants a self-reliant, maximum producing, harmonious team. It is for the doctor who wants to do more than 'make a living,' and wants to *serve* more patients, who wants to provide the highest level of care for his patients, who wants to create a team who will go to battle for him.

If this is you, then this just might be the most powerful book you read this year. This book is about real-world solutions for very common challenges and frustrations that are facing dentistry today.

Many doctors realize that there needs to be change in their hygiene department, but sometimes it sounds easier than it actually is. Humans naturally resist change. We like to stay where we are comfortable. Hygienists can be especially resistant to change – but it doesn't have to be that way! I believe that almost all of that resistance to change stems from 2 things; **Miscommunication** and **Misunderstandings**.

My goal in this book is to break down both the miscommunications and misunderstandings that so many doctors and practices struggle with. These issues can keep you from providing patients with a World-Class dental experience and from realizing profitable practices.

Woody Oakes, Founder of Excellence in Dentistry and publisher of *The Profitable Dentist* has called me "*The world's most famous hygienist.*" If you have ever met me, you know that I am an average hygienist from Salt Lake City, Utah. My family has always come first in my life, and I am the proud mom to 4 wonderful kids and 1 incredible (and highly spoiled) grandchild. My husband has always been my rock and my biggest supporter.

While the road has not always been easy, I knew from very early on that dentistry was where I wanted to be. My first job, while I was still in high school was as an assistant in a dental office. After that I left dentistry for a brief time, even turning down a scholarship to dental hygiene school and thinking that I wanted to study linguistics in college...I realized later that dentistry was my future, and I had made a mistake in turning down that scholarship.

It took me a few years to figure out that linguistics wasn't for me and that my heart was in serving patients and working in the dental field.

Now, without a scholarship and newly married, I applied to dental hygiene school. Shortly after receiving my acceptance I found out I was pregnant with my first child. All of my instructors told me there was no way I could complete hygiene school with a newborn so I set out to prove them all wrong.

I was the top performer in my class, awarded the Sigma Phi Alpha award for academics, and graduated with not only a baby but pregnant with my second child. I knew that I had found my passion, and I couldn't wait to start working.

With 2 young children at home, I quickly recognized that I didn't want to spend all week at work – every hour I was working meant another hour that I was away from my family.

So I started to study other providers to figure out how I could be the most productive with the time I was at work. I wanted to ensure that every minute or every hour that I was away from my family I was providing the highest level of income for them. It didn't take long before I was able to earn what I had previously earned in 4 days in just 2 short days.

God blessed me with 2 more children, and I was able to help provide for our family while only working 10 days a month. While pregnant with my fourth child, the owner of the practice where I had been so successful became ill and decided to sell his practice.

While determining where my future was going, I did some temporary work with practices in the area. I quickly saw that not everybody practiced hygiene the way I did, and both the doctors and the hygienists in these practices all wanted to learn my secrets.

Every day that I was in a practice, I had a goal; I wanted to pay my salary in extra services. Now, often these services weren't a part of the practice's usual protocol and as a result, our production on these days would be really high. I would try to do at least $300 worth of fluoride or $300 worth of sealants to pay my salary. I wanted my salary to be paid in extra services, because I believed in the service AND because I knew what it meant to the doctor to be profitable.

Many of these practices were losing money in hygiene; a lot of experts in dentistry were saying that was how it worked – that it didn't matter if hygiene was productive because hygiene only existed to send restorative work to the doctor's chair. I always felt that if hygiene served as a loss leader, then it's really the patients who are being shorted. When hygiene productivity is low, it often means that patients aren't receiving beneficial preventive care.

Just about every practice I had been a substitute in asked me to come in and work for them as the Hygiene Team Leader and teach the other hygienists in their practice how to do what I was able to do. I kept saying "no" until I realized that I could say "while I can't come work for you, I can teach your hygienists to do what I do" and that's how Hygiene Diamonds was started.

Now, 15 years later, I have helped over 3,712 practices use these ideas to serve their patients at a higher level while driving hygiene profitability, driving more pre-sold restorative work to the dentist's chair, and building a bond with patients so they never want to leave.

I have a lot of dentists and hygienists reach out that say, "We're frustrated because it seems like the things that used to work well for us in our practice and in our community just aren't having the same impact today."

When I began to study the outliers in our profession, I found some really interesting commonalities. The Elite practices, those that are performing far above the average, all have embraced the changes that have come. These high performers don't' resist change, they have developed and embraced a different strategy or different approach for the challenges in dentistry today.

My team visits a lot of dental practices. We find that some practices are clinging to an outdated model of dentistry and are really struggling to succeed. The fee-for-service practice is a rarity today. I'm not saying that this model is not a wonderful thing. If you're a dentist and are succeeding in that model, for heaven's sake, don't change anything. However, I would suggest that the fee-for-service practice that doesn't take insurance is more rare than one might think.

We're seeing a lot of practices - because of changes in the marketplace and changes in what patients are demanding - having to accept insurance and learn how to work with that model. There are advantages and disadvantages with accepting insurance.

Practices that have adapted to the changes in our industry and society are flourishing! These Hygiene-Driven practices are no longer solely reliant on new patients for growth. They have less cancellations and no-shows; there is less stress on doctor and the entire team. They have systems that help them to function as a harmonious team, and the doctor has experienced the lift that comes when the practice profitability is no longer all on their shoulders.

But sadly, the idea of hygiene as a loss leader remains highly prevalent. There are still a lot of people who think that it doesn't matter what you do in hygiene because all they need is one $40,000 case a month. The hygiene production itself is irrelevant if we are just looking for a full-mouth restorative case.

While I understand that there are some places in the country and some truly unique providers where this model can work – the reality of today's dentistry is bread-and-butter dentistry. This is what patients are asking for, and it's what patients are accepting.

For me, it's not as much whether or not you can find the $40,000 cases, but to completely disregard the valuable services that hygienists provide to patients every day, in my book, is neglecting your patient. Preventative services matter.

If a practice is low in hygiene production, in my opinion, their patients are not being served at a level that they deserve.

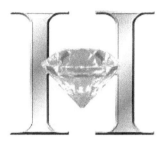

Chapter 2

Why Hygienists Are Special

While every position in your practice is important and every team member is special, hygienists are a rare hybrid of team member and producer and provide your practice with incredible opportunity.

Hygienists have the biggest opportunity, of just about everyone in the practice, to build a relationship with patients. As a producer, they can produce revenue for the practice, which differentiates them from other team members.

We can't do what we do without our teams and recognize they are valuable too; however, they are not producers. An assistant is in a supportive role; a front desk person is also in a support role. They don't personally add to the production and the revenue of a practice – they support it.

Hygienists have a large impact on our ability to retain patients at a higher level. I can't tell you how many times over the years patients will say, "I love coming and seeing my hygienist. She's the best!" Many times our patients become like members of our family.

In many patients' minds, they develop a bond, a long-term relationship with a hygienist that in some ways can become more powerful than the relationship with the dentist because they spend more time with the hygienist.

Especially when we are highly focused on patient care and providing an incredible experience, our patients feel the difference! Part of what makes a hygienist special is when they go above and beyond to really show that they care for the patient.

Taking the time to have risk assessment conversations, discussing and setting goals that patients have for their future health, this is what sets a World Class Hygienist apart from the masses. Becoming invested in their success and giving them guidance and support, this is the way that hygienists show they truly care.

The hygienists that have more of a struggle are those that view their role as more of a lecturer. When we lecture or shame our patients and tell them what they're not doing with home care… patients don't feel the positive emotions that inspire long-term relationships. Believe it or not, there are many hygienists that feel it is their responsibility to shame patients into better home care. We have found that doesn't help a practice grow in the long run.

World Class Hygienists are those that have become partners with their patients and are helping them achieve a higher level of health. Minimizing cavities, minimizing infection, trying to avoid future problems, and helping them know what they can do differently to achieve better results, this is what creates long-time patients who refer as well as increased case acceptance!

When we see bleeding gums, we used to think, "They need to improve their home care; they need to floss." Well, now, it's a much different conversation. We look at their health overall, what does that look like? How well are they doing at home? Do they need better tools? Do we need to get them anti-microbials that can help reduce the bacterial load in their mouth? There are a lot of other elements involved in the health of the tissue that we need to evaluate and that patients need to understand.

Patients do not respond well to the shaming, the guilt-tripping, and the lecturing of the past. They aren't telling you they want out; they are just quietly leaving, choosing another practice and not referring anyone to yours. The challenge is – you may never know why this patient left.

You might be asking... is it dangerous for me to see my patients develop such a high bond with a hygienist who could leave my practice at any time?

Well, yes and no, right?

We want patients to feel connected with their hygienist. We want the partnership to develop, but we are striving for a healthy relationship. We also need to be sure that we are managing these relationships appropriately.

There are hygienists who feel like they own their patients, that if they take a day off they don't want anyone else seeing *their* patients We want the relationship between our patients and their hygiene provider to be strong, but also healthy for the practice.

When we have hygienists becoming territorial, this is not a patient friendly strategy. Patients are the most important element in any practice, and often our core values support caring for the patient in the best possible way. When we allow hygienists to control "their" patients in this way, the relationship is no longer healthy.

That is not the approach we want. That doesn't benefit the doctor, the practice, or the patient. The patients belong to the practice, not the hygienist.

Which is why we need to create more solid relationships with other team members as well, not just the hygienist.

As the doctor, you should be conducting an emotionally connected new patient exam, which starts an important bond with you. Your financial team should be conducting emotionally connected financial arrangements, so that patients create a bond with them.

This way we are all cultivating important relationships with the patients, and they feel connected to your entire team.

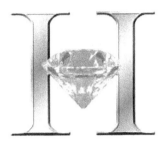

CHAPTER 3

The Current Model of Hygiene is Broken …

There are really only 2 ways to increase revenue. You can either increase the number of patient encounters or you can increase the production per encounter.

If you are thinking of shortening your hygiene appointment times – DON'T. It is much easier and more beneficial for your patients and your practice to increase the production per encounter.

Many dentists have been told that the solution to increasing hygiene production is to shorten the time for each hygiene appointment. Hygienists are then asked to provide world-class services in just 30-40-45 minute appointment times. The shortening of appointment times is an adaptive strategy designed to drive revenue by increasing volume. I call this Accelerated Hygiene.

Increasing patient encounters in this way does equal an increase in production. However, it also equals other less desirable things. It equals **less referrals from existing patients** and **an increase in broken appointments.** It also often equals **increased errors**, from missed steps.

I understand the desire to see an increase in hygiene productivity – it's what I teach daily. However, many practices have offers that dramatically reduce hygiene productivity. New Patient specials are very common, and hygiene takes the hit. Hygiene has long been the "Loss Leader" in dentistry.

The Loss Leader Strategy: Hygiene services are offered at a discounted rate in the *hopes* of attracting new patients. Then once the new patient is in the chair for the discounted hygiene service, the *hope* that they accept restorative services - which will then help the practice to grow.

While this strategy does succeed when done right,

with all the changes in dental insurance and the need to participate in varying levels of PPOs and the reduction in reimbursements from the insurance companies, it has become much harder to remain profitable in hygiene.

To keep the practice in the black, some teach that hygiene appointments especially for "New Patient Specials" have to be shorter. More patients during the day ensure more revenue.

The flaw in this structure is that it is impossible to provide a world-class level of care in hygiene in a 45-minute-or-less appointment time. I have even seen practices that expect the hygienist to do everything for a preventive care visit in just 30 minutes **without an assistant.**

For many hygienists, even experienced and talented practitioners, getting everything done well in a 30 minute appointment time is next to impossible. Providing a positive patient experience and completing the standard of care in this amount of time is just not realistic.

In my opinion, this is like expecting a molar root canal and crown preparation to be done in 30 minutes. Even highly skilled dentists recognize there are too many steps to be done during the process to accomplish everything and still have a quality root canal and crown when finished.

While this example is not entirely accurate, as we are comparing apples and oranges, the concept of trying to provide quality in an unreasonably short time frame is similar.

Sadly, there are many practice management consultants working within dentistry today that advocate for shortening hygiene appointments to impractical lengths. Interestingly enough, many of these consultants are not clinicians and, therefore, have never attempted to treat a patient in this shortened time period.

On a side note, if you feel you must increase the number of patient encounters, I suggest moving to an Assisted Model of Hygiene. When done correctly, you will be able to increase the number of encounters while still providing the time and care needed for each patient. That is another example of an adaptive strategy that can revolutionize hygiene, but caution! This also needs to be done right and can fail when not implemented carefully. That is another topic for another time.

With all of this being said, a **change to hygiene is needed**. The current model of losing revenue in hygiene is not sustainable. My experience would suggest that the strategy of quantity over quality is flawed. I prefer an adaptive strategy that focuses on complete care.

The other option of increasing production per encounter has proven to be the better strategy. I have found that there are 3 benefits that the practice experiences when they focus on quality over quantity:

1. A more productive visit resulting in higher overall hygiene revenue

2. A reduction in cancellations, no-shows, and open time in the hygiene schedule because of the value built for future appointments

3. An increase in referrals to the practice due to the exceptional experience and personalized care

The most important benefit that I see is that patients that go through hygiene under this system have a deeper connection with the hygiene provider and the practice. They feel better served, which results in more restorative dentistry; even more cosmetic and implant dentistry coming out of hygiene.

Are you currently satisfied with the level at which your practice is educating and communicating treatment with your patients?

The Role of the Hygienist is Changing
Hygiene is changing rapidly right now! We used to be defined as the ones who kept teeth clean so they could be restored. Now, we bring so much more to the table; it is both exciting and overwhelming at the

same time. If we want to become more effective with increasing production per encounter, I have defined three roles that a hygienist must utilize to maximize their impact in a practice:

3 Key Roles of a World Class Hygiene Provider

Preventive Therapist: As the "preventive therapist" the hygienist becomes the source of information regarding the menu of preventive services. When we use the full menu of preventative services (regardless of age and insurance) we are in fact, providing a much higher level of patient care and a level of care that our patients want and need.

Periodontal Therapist: It's not just about saving teeth anymore; it's now about saving lives. Patients are at much greater risk of other serious medical disorders if we do not address their periodontal health – and this starts while in the hygiene chair.

Patient Treatment Advocate: I mentioned earlier that the backbone of the dental practice is the hygienist. This is why; I define 'Patient Treatment Advocate' as a key role. This key role is responsible for moving restorative dentistry onto the doctor's side. When we maximize this role, we see case acceptance skyrocket.

Let's look at each one more closely….

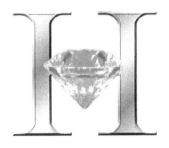

CHAPTER 4

How to Maximize the Role of Preventative Therapist

People like to be involved in decisions regarding their health, and their dental health is no different. Gone are the days of 'lecturing' and 'scolding.' Patients have choices, and they are not afraid to go elsewhere.

Our job as a Hygiene provider should be to advocate for the dental health of our patients. In doing so, we also provide the dental practice with maximum potential for revenue.

Our goal is to serve all patients at the highest level and the high production naturally follows. But as a business owner, **I know that what is measured and managed will improve**. So here are 3 key metrics that I look at for this role:

1. Adult Fluoride Acceptance Rate: Most practices have a fluoride acceptance rate under 10%. You should have a minimum of 80%; most of the practices that we work with see 90%-95% acceptance of adult fluoride treatments.

2. Sealant Acceptance Rate: Regardless of age or insurance, if the tooth would benefit from a sealant, that is what should be presented to the patient. How often are we placing sealants? A goal for many or our members is just 4 sealants/day

3. Bonded Desensitizing Acceptance Rate: If more than 85% of all adults complain of sensitive teeth, we should be taking the opportunity to provide a bonded agent that will both seal and protect the vulnerable Class V area where recession has occurred.

What is the best way to maximize the acceptance of these procedures? We need to work to engage our patients and walk them through their personal situation. Many are frustrated at the level of decay they experience or at the frequency of cavities they have even though they are working hard at home.

The more we can involve them in the conversation and have them truly understand the risks and benefits, the higher acceptance rate we will have when presenting solutions.

It all starts with how we set up the visit. At every opportunity possible, we want to engage our patients in high level conversations.

What do I mean by this? Take, for example, probing. It's a vital part of our exam, but have you maximized the potential of the process?

I start all of my tissue health assessments, or periodontal probing, with a conversation designed to help the patient know what I am looking for.

"I am going to check your tissues for infection. This helps us detect any problems or disease in your gums. You will hear me saying a series of numbers for each tooth, and Chelsea is going to record the findings for us. A 1-3 means that the tissue is healthy. A 4 means there is infection. A 5 indicates that the infection has already spread to the bone."

Why would I do this? Because now the patient is hearing my exam, and when they hear 4 and 5's they immediately ask, *"What do we need to do to take care of that?"*

And now, when I explain that we need to do periodontal therapy, they have the proof to back that up, and were already in the mind-set that we need to do something different.

They are coming to us looking for a solution, where as before (without this knowledge) they felt that we were just trying to 'sell' them something they didn't need.

These conversations matter! It is critical that we have a system and a script to follow to drive acceptance for every service that we provide in hygiene.

Let's take a look at fluoride:

92% of Dentists are getting less than 74% acceptance with adult fluoride

Most often fluoride is presented something like this (if at all),

"We should probably talk about a fluoride treatment,

but it isn't covered by your insurance."

This doesn't inspire anyone to accept this service. When we simply change our language and use these 3 specific steps for presenting fluoride, we drive the acceptance rate through the roof:

Step #1: New research has shown _____

The first part is really important, especially for hygienists that aren't currently offering fluoride consistently to adults.

Many practices routinely use fluoride with children because that is when insurance will pay for it. Too often, we don't give our adult patients compelling enough reasons to do fluoride, and we may not even offer it at all.

If you are trying to offer fluoride to adults now and you haven't in the past, I have found the best way is to start by saying *"New research shows."*

This is critical for those practices that have not offered fluoride as a part of the preventive care appointment.

"New research shows that for patients who consistently have a professionally applied fluoride

treatment, we can see up to 75% fewer new cavities. This is huge for patients who are always struggling with decay."

Step #2: Here is why fluoride would be good for you today _____

The second step is to share with the patient specific reasons that you feel fluoride would benefit them.

The more specific you can be about what you see in their mouth the better! If they have exposed root surfaces and dry mouth, they are at a very high risk for decay.

We know how vulnerable those areas are; we need to bring that to their attention.

If they have crown margins, large fillings, or many restorations, talk about how fluoride can help protect their investment.

They have spent money and time in rebuilding their mouth, and fluoride will help prevent recurrent decay and failure of their dental work.

Step #3: Bad news, insurance won't help with the cost – Good news, it's only $XX

The third step is to let the patient know that there is

both good news and bad news about fluoride.

Their dental insurance company will not help with the cost. That is the bad news.

The good news is that topical application of fluoride is very affordable. It is not an expensive procedure, especially when compared with crowns and other restorations.

Many patients see that investing in fluoride even if it's an out-of-pocket expense makes good financial sense. We need to help them see the value in investing in topically applied fluoride. So, again, here are the steps for increasing fluoride acceptance:

Step #1: New research has shown _____

Step #2: Here is why fluoride would be good for you today _____

Step #3: Bad news, insurance won't help with the cost – Good news, it's only $XX

Doesn't it sounds better when you say...

"Susan, are you aware that new research has shown that if we do a fluoride varnish every time we polish your teeth, that we can reduce future

cavities? We can minimize future decay by as much as 75%. Earlier you mentioned that you were frustrated with always having problems with your teeth. Let's turn that around. Fluoride varnish can help us do that."

Below is a copy of the flowchart I created for our clients to remember the 3 steps:

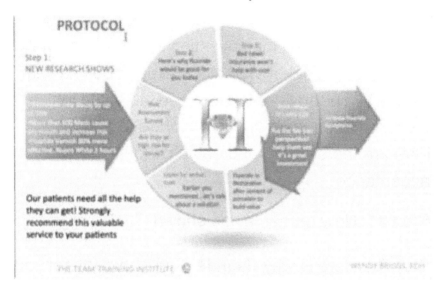

"Everyone has a 95% chance of experiencing caries in the pits and fissures of their teeth if sealants aren't used in those areas."- ADA

Sealants are a service that many people would like if given the opportunity. We see adults get excited about sealants; they just haven't been offered them before. Why is this?

We know that early stage cavities and incipient decay are stopped by sealants. But many dentists have been hesitant to recommend sealants consistently because the early sealant materials had high failure rates. This is because the products themselves were not nearly as good and our procedures were not nearly as good as they are today.

We now have caries detection technology. We have many lasers that help detect decay: DIAGNOdent, Spectra, Soprocare cameras and even the CariVu. As technology continues to improve, we will have even better tools to aid us in detection of decay.

A few years ago, we wouldn't have thought of doing a sealant on an adult, but with the challenges that we are seeing in patients today it's a viable option. We see medications that cause xerostomia. High risk patients also have other risk factors. With the enhancement of the technology we are now able to make a more educated determination of which teeth would be good candidates for sealants.

Our standard of care is now to recommend sealants on all posterior teeth, NOT just those that insurance will pay for. Insurance companies only pay for sealants on children, but that doesn't mean that sealants don't benefit adults.

Dr. David Gore a prosthodontist and the director of the restorative dentistry department at the University of Kentucky, said that for "adults age 40 and over sealants may be the treatment of choice" because of rapidly changing medical conditions.

There was also a longevity study completed by Simonsen that said a one-time placement of a sealant could provide a benefit for 15 years. After 15 years there is a 54% reduction in decay. If you place a sealant and monitor it and maintain it, it can reduce decay by 74% over that 15-year period.

This new research has many dentists rethinking how they are utilizing sealants. When good protocol is used, combined with the latest technology, sealants can be a valuable procedure for all ages.

I often challenge hygienists to find at least four sealants a day in their practice. If a hygienist were to place four sealants on average every day, this adds up to a hefty amount of increased productivity. Not to mention the number of teeth we are protecting each day!

This is why I love to help grow practices. We find

ways that they can serve their patients at a higher level while increasing productivity and profitability.

Everyone wins.

When we change our sealant approach, we also stress the value of doing same-day sealants. Patients of today are looking for convenience, and the more often we can provide that for them the more successful we will be.

Over 80% of the adult population suffers from sensitive teeth,

Hypersensitivity affects 45 million adults in the US alone.

However, in many dental practices we don't consistently offer a bonded solution for someone with sensitive teeth.

This is most likely because many of the products we have used in the past didn't last long term.

Many of our desensitizing agents were designed to go underneath a restoration. When acting as a stand-alone desensitizer, they didn't last long enough for us to justify the fee.

Now we have several exciting options that we can use that are proven to provide a benefit for up to three years.

Our extremely sensitive patients really appreciate us solving this problem for them.

The bonded service also protects that vulnerable area from decay, giving the patient the double benefit of no more pain and protection.

When desensitizing agents are presented in the right frame, we have an 89.9% acceptance rate. The script that I use for this level of acceptance is as follows:

"We have an exciting new service that can help immediately remove the pain and discomfort from your sensitive tooth. It also protects it over time. It's actually easier if I show you how it works rather than try to explain to you how it works. Let's do this, we can try it on your most sensitive tooth. If it doesn't work, you don't pay. If it does work, it's only $29."

I have yet to write off a treatment. Now, the key ... once I have applied the treatment, I then say,

"If you start to notice sensitivity creeping back, most likely you have had more recession in the area."

I have opened the loop and started the conversation in their mind, that if they start to feel sensitivity again, they are likely experiencing additional recession. This is key for future treatment and future treatment acceptance.

It's not what you say ... it's how you say it.

Framing your conversations so that the benefit to the patients are crystal clear. And ensuring that everyone in your office, this includes; the hygienists, the financial coordinator, the front desk team, and even the doctor, are in agreement and following the same script when offering any service will be the key to your success.

So what can maximizing this role do for your practice? Let's take a look at some conservative numbers; let's say you add:

- 8 Fluoride treatments a day at $25 = $3,200 a month and $38,400 a year

- 4 sealants a day at $45 = $2,880 a month and $34,560 a year

- 4 desensitizing agents a day at $39 = $2,496 a month and $29,952 a year

Combined that is a potential $102,912 PER

HYGIENIST increase in hygiene production – and just utilizing the 3 key metrics in the preventative therapist role.

One of the best tools I use to build value for preventive services is CAMBRA. Caries Management by Risk Assessment.

The ADA has been recommending that we treat all patients utilizing this for some time now, but most practices don't.

It really is challenging to find the time to do everything there is to do.

Many practices don't have a system in place for doing risk assessment. We know how important this is, but the ADA's survey is three pages long!

Dentists and hygienists alike get excited when I share the tool I use to facilitate the risk assessment conversation in dental practices in just 90 seconds. (And I'll share it with you in just a few pages.)

How at Risk are Your Patients?

You might be surprised! It is often stunning when we look at the amount of sugar and the PH levels in the drinks that are common amongst patients.

Product	ACID PH LOW=Bad	SUGAR per 12 oz
Pure Water	7.00 Neutral	0
Dasani Water/ Aquafina Water	3.0 5.0	0
Diet Coke	3.39	
Red Wine	3.3	0
Mountain Dew	3.22	11.0 tsp
Gatorade	2.95	3.3 tsp
Pepsi	2.49	9.8 tsp
Coke	2.63	9.3 tsp

Even those that are choosing water, will be surprised at the PH levels of today's bottled water.

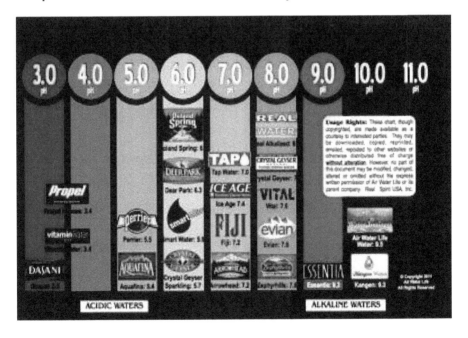

What constitutes "high risk" for adult patients?

The ADA defines "high risk" as:

- 3 or more lesions in the last 3 years

- Suboptimal fluoride exposure

- Xerostomia or Dry Mouth

- Have multiple factors that may increase caries risk

In addition, we have to be aware of the additional items that may increase patients' caries risk. Things like....

- High titers of cariogenic bacteria

- Prolonged nursing (bottle or breast)

- Development of or acquired enamel defects

- Multi-surface restorations

- Chemo/radiation therapy

- Eating disorders

- Cariogenic diet

- Active orthodontic treatment

- Restoration overhangs and open margins

- Plus many more

When we have a risk assessment conversation with patients and use the brochure below, it's like putting prevention on steroids. Most patients don't SEE a need for the preventative services, and it's our job to SHOW them the need, and this does exactly that.

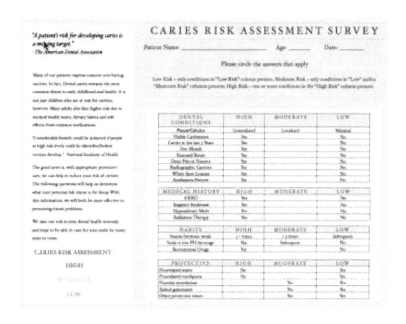

In using a tool like this, the conversation can take place in 90 seconds or less! Without using a tool like this, it takes 3x as a long if it happens at all.

AND now, if we have CAMBRA documentation, we are able to submit and possibly even receive payment from insurance companies at a greater level.

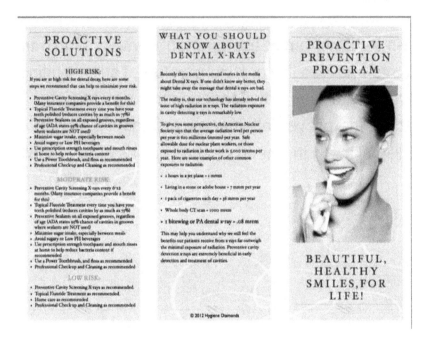

To download a FREE copy of this brochure and access my FREE training on how this one tool accounts for 90% of my case acceptance and how I can do it all in 90 seconds or less go to:

www.HygieneDiamonds.com/risk-assessment

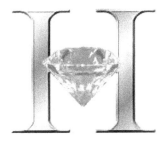

CHAPTER 5

How to Maximize the Role of Periodontal Therapist

The second role of the hygienist is that of a Periodontal Therapist.

Many consultants and hygiene educators focus heavily on periodontal therapy, as it is a critical component in the life of a dental hygienist.

However, it is not uncommon to see a practice that is still treating periodontal infection today with the same strategies and technology that they were using 5 years ago. Sometimes even 10 years ago.

This is truly alarming! Many things have changed. We have better tools, better science about what causes periodontal infection, and how to drastically reduce it. We know so much more about the Oral-Systemic link, and serious health risks that exist with the presence of inflammation in the body.

We have laser techniques, Oral DNA testing methods, better home care products, and additional resources like Arestin and other adjunctive options for patients.

If we are truly maximizing potential in our role as a Periodontal Therapist, we are seeing periodontal disease, talking about it, and treating it.

We should have extremely high acceptance rates for these advanced services; supervised neglect is not an option.

We discuss Periodontal Disease with existing patients as well as new patients, and we are treating it with every available weapon in our arsenal.

I review hundreds of Practice Analysis reports every year as a recommended consulting partner for Henry Schein Dental. I am asked to evaluate how periodontal services are being performed, and it is stunning to see how often our perception of how perio is being treated is so different from the reality!

When most dentists are asked what percentage of their patients should be receiving periodontal care, they will respond 25% or even 40%.

When we look at actual utilization of these codes, the reality is that only 1.9% of their patients received periodontal care in the last year.

My take on this is ... I don't believe that we are not recognizing and discussing the care that patients need. I believe that the patients don't understand the need and therefore are not moving forward with treatment.

I use a simple approach to gaining a higher level of acceptance for Periodontal Services. I talk about utilizing technology to provide a measure of proof.

Use your intra-oral cameras, especially the incredible Perio Mode feature available on the Soprocare camera. (My new favorite!) to help the patient see for themselves what is happening in their mouth.

I then follow up with 3 simple things we need to

do to treat the infection in their mouth.

"To clear up this infection, we need to do these 3 things...."

I then go on to explain the 3 steps needed to clear up the infection:

#1: *"We need to do a deep, more aggressive cleaning than you've had in the past."* And then I stop...

At this point the patient is probably thinking this is going to involve pain and discomfort so we need to reassure them we will do everything possible to keep them comfortable.

Explain that we have advanced technology that enables us to be incredibly effective in dealing with the bacteria, without pain.

I have found the best analogy that help patients understand what needs to be done is when I make a comparison with a splinter.

You can explain it's like having a splinter under the skin. *"If we don't get rid of the splinter, you're never going to heal. In the same way, we need to do the cleaning to get the buildup out and to clear the area of bacteria".*

If a patient has not been in for some time, this helps to explain why more action is needed than a 'standard' cleaning. They need to catch up.

#2: *"We need to change a few things that you are doing at home."* You have to be very careful here - It's been proven that nobody likes to get a lecture on what they are not doing.

So we need to position this carefully. We may suggest they use a prescription mouthwash daily to help keep the bacteria under control.

They are often open to this, and people are willing to use what we recommend if they truly believe we believe it will help them.

It can also help to recommend using a power toothbrush. When it comes to recommending the power brush, I often use the analogy of a screwdriver – a basic job can be done with a manual screwdriver, but a big job will need a power screwdriver.

With the level of infection they have in their mouth, it requires a tool that will do more for them. "*In the same way, the infection that has built up in your mouth means you need a power brush to get rid of it. We need something that can do more for you than a basic manual toothbrush."*

When introducing the idea of a power brush, it can be useful to say: *"We don't care where you get it as long as you get one."*

You can suggest that high-end brushes such as Sonicare or Oral B have been found to be more effective than manual brushing and add:

"We carry them, here in the office, because we know you are busy and we try to make everything as easy for you as possible. Plus, we can provide them for you at a cost less than you would pay at WalMart."

The patient then understands we're not just trying to push a sale; we're trying to give them the tools they need to be more effective against the infection.

#3: *"We need to see you back more often."*

We know how important it is for the patients to come in for three or four-month recall visits, but patients don't realize how critical it is. They are only used to hearing that they need to have their teeth cleaned every 6 months.

They don't know that bacteria has been proven to regenerate in just 21-60 days after scaling and root planing – and that they can have reinfection and more bleeding within that time.

Patients really appreciate when we simplify things for them, so it often helps to use the 'oil change' analogy.

We explain that after the deep cleaning, they are starting with a clean slate but if they don't come back more often – they may end up back where they started.

The disease can reoccur, and the infection spirals out of control and we lose ground.

We explain that it's like buying a brand-new car – it won't last very long if you don't change the oil regularly.

So, to maximize healing, we need to see them back more often than they may have come in the past.

The latest research helps us to understand that maximizing our role as a periodontal therapist is not just about saving teeth, it really is about saving lives.

We know that dental health affects overall health, but patients do not. There's compelling scientific proof that dental health affects overall health – for example, people with periodontal disease are at greater risk of heart disease.

The National Institute of Health states,

"Oral bacteria shed from chronic periodontal infections enter the circulatory system and may contribute to diseases of the heart and other organs.

The role of periodontal diseases in causing or contributing to other serious conditions is the subject of ongoing laboratory and clinical research.

"As this research unfolds in the coming years, it may be that a trip to the dentist not only could have benefits for your oral health but also help reduce your chances of developing related systemic conditions."

Scientists now know that the bacteria in our mouths exist as a complex, multilayered community called oral biofilm.

Scientists already are in the process of dissecting the dynamics of these bacterial communities. This research may give dentists and hygienists the tools to target their treatment specifically to the bacteria that trigger periodontal disease.

We are already seeing this with laser procedures specifically targeting diseased tissues.

This is why for us to truly maximize our role as a periodontal therapist, we need constant refreshers. We MUST keep our protocol and our techniques up to date in this critical area.

If you haven't embraced new technology or made any critical changes to your periodontal program in a few years, it is time to take a hard look at doing this now.

Wendy Briggs

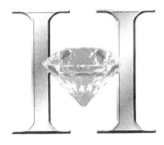

CHAPTER 6

How to Maximize the Role of the Patient Treatment Advocate

The third role is that of a Patient Treatment Advocate. Hygienists often underestimate what a critical role we have in helping our patients make choices about the dentistry they need.

How many times have they turned to the hygienist or another clinical team member to ask, "Do I really need to have this done?" or "How long can I wait before I get this taken care of?"

The reality is, patients do want the team's opinion

and recommendations when it comes to the choices they have about treatment.

Did you know that 65% of all production completed in the Restorative Department in a dental practice is referred from hygiene?

If this is true, I often wonder why so many dentists feel like they could use more personal help in this area.

What tools do you have for aiding you in case presentation?

Are you consistently using them?

How involved is the hygiene team in this effort?

The old paradigm for case presentation is to educate, educate, educate. Although I do think educating the patient is important, we have to remember to keep things simple. We often think that education means we have to teach them dentistry. We think they need to know how to do the procedure in order to accept it. This causes us to use words the patient doesn't understand.

When we use complicated terminology, the patient often ends up being confused. This is the last thing we want! Confused patients are unable to make a decision about treatment.

Do you ever hear, "I want to get it taken care of, but I need to go home and check with my spouse?"

Patients needing to check their schedules call their insurance, or any other number of excuses, are most likely confused about recommendations, overwhelmed, or both!

This leads to frustration. These 3 emotions are usually behind case acceptance failures, and we must avoid them at all costs: Confusion, Overwhelm, and Frustration.

Our challenge, then, is to approach case presentation with the new paradigm. I have several key rules that if followed can help you explode your Case Acceptance.

Rule #1: Simplify! Talk in terms your patients understand. Often it's not what you say, but how you say it. In Case Acceptance, what THEY SEE is so much more important than what YOU SAY!

This is why I love to use my tools! There are several

things I can't live without when talking with patients about opportunity for treatment in their mouths.

• <u>DIAGNOdent,</u> or any kind of "Cavity Detecting Laser," helps patients see the proof of a problem for themselves. They hear the alarm signal, they see the number (I have the patient hold it so they can participate) and they know without me having to say anything that there is a potential problem. Follow this up with another powerful tool: your intra-oral camera. Show them exactly what that reading of 34 looks like and why you are concerned.

• <u>Intra-Oral Camera</u>, again, the value of this tool is that the patients can see for themselves. A cracked tooth in the mouth and a cracked tooth up on the monitor or television look like two different things. I prefer my patients see it as big as life on the screen. This way, there is urgency without me having to create it for them.. The images from the camera take away any doubts the patient may have about their mouth.

"Seeing is Believing" is what it's all about!

Comments from the patient prove how powerful the camera is. I can't tell the patient that their teeth look terrible, but once they see it with the camera, often they are the ones that will say, "It looks terrible!"

Many practices have these amazing tools, but they sit collecting dust. Lack of systems, perception that there "just isn't enough time" or lack of confidence on the part of the hygiene team often are the cause of underutilized valuable resources.

Sometimes it may be a problem of poor quality equipment that is difficult to use. Maybe we don't have enough of them, and hygienists are having to track them down or wait their turn.

In reality, once hygienists learn the proper use of these tools, and how presenting opportunities with the right verbal skills actually SAVES time, the more they will use these tools.

If you want more success with case acceptance, dust off the DIAGNOdent, take out that camera, and get going! If you need more of anything, get a commitment from hygiene that they will use it; then just get it done.

Rule #2: Build Value - Patients will find a way to pay for what they WANT. So we should really focus on helping them want to have their teeth taken care of.

Why should they want to have this done?

Why would YOU do it?

Talk about this with your patients! I often will say, "If this was in my mouth, this is what I would do to fix it." They are looking to us for guidance. They value and want your opinion.

So, to be more effective when talking with patients about what they need, don't be afraid to tell them what you would do. We should focus more often on what the direct benefits are.

Instead of telling the patient how we place implants, tell them the benefits of having them.

"When we place implants in your mouth, you will be able to chew without pain, almost like natural teeth. There will be nothing to take out and clean; you will be able to brush and floss these teeth as you did before. By the way, have I told you that implants have porcelain crowns on them that look incredibly like natural teeth?"

Building Value while keeping things simple can revolutionize your acceptance. Avoid the natural tendency to make things too complicated. Focus on the benefits for the patient, and they will be interested in learning more.

You will be amazed at what your patients accept when they understand what you are recommending, and WANT to have it done!

To find out where your practice currently stands, download our **Rate Your Hygiene Performance Worksheet at** www.HygieneDiamonds.com/rate-hygiene

Wendy Briggs

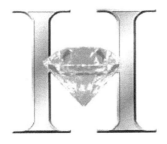

CHAPTER 7

How to Increase Case Acceptance Using Tribal Language

Clear Diagnostic Criteria: There are many practices who don't communicate their standard protocol for diagnosing dentistry. As hygienists, we obviously don't diagnose, but we should have clear guidelines for what our doctors would do in a variety of situations. Not having this makes the hygienists' job very difficult... if you were to show the same patient to 10 different dentists, you will likely receive a range of treatment plans from the most productive to the least productive based on each dentist's subjective data and personal treatment planning.

This is to be expected but is not good when the range of treatment is occurring in one office. This lack of consistency hampers your hygienists' ability to help you increase case acceptance.

Dentistry isn't black and white. This is why it is so critical to define the diagnostic and treatment criteria for your practice.

We see a disconnect in this area in many practices. In fact, not only will each dentist have a different opinion on the treatment plan for our patient, if you were to ask each doctor at different times of the day for their diagnosis, you would again have a range of answers. When fresh (i.e. in the morning), some might tend to be more assertive in treatment recommendations. This is when we are often fired up to utilize same-day dentistry skills. As the day wears on and the provider wears down, treatment planning may become a little more conservative... we see dentists willing to 'wait' on some things that we might not have put off in the morning.

Because of this, your practice needs to have criteria

set in place based on where you, the doctor, feel most comfortable treating your patients.

You need to define things like:

- What defines a cavity in your practice? .... What are the radiographic findings that indicate decay?

- What are the criteria for determining that a crown is needed? What are the clinical findings that indicate that a filling will no longer serve as the best option?

- What kind of filling material is your Gold standard? Are there materials you will not use?

- What are the symptoms that indicate that endodontic treatment is needed?

- When is a tooth damaged beyond repair?

- Which tooth replacement is ideal? Should we prepare the patient for an implant or a bridge?

- When do we use a removable prosthesis to replace the teeth?

- When do we use a fixed prosthesis supported by teeth or implants?

- When do we use a removable that's supported by teeth implants and/or tissue?

When you have your criteria spelled out and defined, you give your hygiene team a standard of measurement. This helps ensure that we are not over-diagnosing and not under-diagnosing. Possibly the most important benefit, you can now utilize your entire team in presenting treatment.

Without defined criteria, we often see varying levels of care for your patients depending on which provider they saw that day. This only increases the patient's and the hygienist's level of confusion. If you and your hygienists are not on the same page and are not consistently presenting a solid front to patients, they can lose their trust in you. Without trust, case acceptance becomes very difficult.

We want to ensure that every provider, every team member they see that day is able to provide the patient with the reassurance that the recommended treatment is the best course of treatment.

This can only be accomplished if the entire team

has defined criteria and uses the same language.

We accomplish this 'across team' communication by using what we call 'Tribal Language.' We have found that everything we defined above can be placed into 3 categories:

1. **Mandatory:** These are the most urgent needs and are for problems that involve anything that is broken, infected, or decayed. With mandatory needs, it is imperative that we act quickly or conditions will become worse and more costly. A good analogy is a building that is on fire; we need to get the fire out quickly and efficiently to minimize damage.

2. **Elective:** is something that can cause a future problem if not addressed at some point. This is what used to be our 'watch' list. These issues are those that are starting to cause concern but don't have any active decay. A good example might be fillings that are starting to deteriorate. You wouldn't feel right about saying these have got to be done, but in reality it would be good to replace them before a crisis occurs. A good analogy here is rebuilding or remodeling the house. Sometimes updating outdated restorations with better materials will help us preserve the value long term.

3. **Cosmetic:** is anything that would enhance the appearance of the smile. This also provides the patient with an opportunity to discuss any kind of cosmetic treatment they may be interested in. Having this conversation allows the patient to direct their course of treatment and become engaged in their care.

I suggest that you take an evening to define all of these criteria into these 3 categories, using the worksheet pictured. Then share your ideal guidelines with your team. You may even want to laminate this and place it in your practice manual and every operatory so that everyone has access to your team's tribal language.

Teams that utilize these systems for discussing treatment realize incredible results! Just by using these 3 words, we have seen doctors increase case acceptance by as much as 50%. The important thing to the hygiene team is the confidence that comes by knowing how we can best support our doctors and our patients when discussing ideal care.

To download this worksheet and the definitions to create Mandatory/Elective/Cosmetic languaging in your practice go to:
www.HygieneDiamonds.com/tribal-language

Having your team preassess using your diagnostic criteria is not only helpful, but becomes a critical and often overlooked step in case presentation and case acceptance. This is the piece of the puzzle that allows for same-day dentistry.

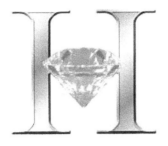

CHAPTER 8

5 Keys to Sustainable Success in Hygiene

Once we focus on maximizing the 3 roles of hygiene, we see how valuable these systems can be to the growth of the practice. There are other systems that are also powerful, if we want to see these initial results sustained over the long term. Over the years, I have identified 5 keys to sustainable success in hygiene. The first one is…

Key #1: Systems for a consistent world-class experience

For every 10,000 organizations, 2,000 actually

develop goals. 400 outline a plan to achieve those goals. 80 act on their plan, while only16 check their progress on the goals they have set. It is stunning to know that only 3 to 4 create systems for each goal-related task. Do you have systems?

Warning: Most practices THINK that they have a system ... but a system is defined as having 4 components:

1. The Commander's Intent: Why is a system important and what is the purpose of this system? We need to identify the ideal outcome.

2. Flowchart: Showing the different steps of the system and who is responsible for each step is a critical component.

3. Scripts: Define the communication expected and how we want the process to happen consistently.

4. Follow-up Mechanism: This is vital to create checks and balances and ensure that the system is implemented. These need to be a part of the daily/weekly/monthly routine.

So what should you have a system for? Everything you want done well! We have identified a minimum of 75 systems that are necessary for a successful dental practice. Systems are needed for consistency in everything from room setup, to order and process of each procedure, for utilization of materials, to what the doctor wants to be able to delegate to the clinical assistants... We need systems for ordering, hiring and training, marketing, keeping the schedule full, room setup and breakdown, sterilization, and the list goes on and on. A few examples are:

- Perio-Health Maintenance
- 6-Point Probing
- Hygiene Services: Fluoride, Sealant, Desensitizing Treatment, & Radiograph Protocols
- Crown & Bridge Protocol
- Sedation Protocol
- Root Canal Protocol
- Caries Detection Protocol
- Risk Assessment Protocol
- Intra-oral Camera Protocol
- Handoffs to Drive Case Acceptance
- Clinical Note & Charting and Documentation Protocol
- Cavity Detecting Laser Protocol
- Oral Cancer Screening Protocol
- World-Class Exam Protocol

Let's look closer at a few examples of elements of a Hygiene System:

Hygiene Recall Appointments
Checklist of Non-Negotiable & Negotiable Clinical Elements

Non-Negotiable

_____ Health HX Review/Update
    _____Medications
    _____Allergies
    _____Surgeries/Illnesses/Diseases/Conditions/Blood Transfusions/Tobacco
_____ Radiographs: Anterior PAs
    _____Missing Teeth
    _____Endodontically-Treated Teeth
    _____Implant-Replaced Teeth
    _____Existing Restorations
_____ Radiographs: Periodic
    _____Bitewings
    _____FMX
_____ DIAGNOdent Screening
_____ Intra-oral Photos: Clinical Conditions
    _____Cracks
    _____Large Amalgams
    _____Anterior/Cosmetic Restorations (Veneers, Crowns, etc.)

_____ Perio Charting
_____ Prophylaxis
    _____Scale, Polish, and Floss
    _____Other Scheduled Procedures (Fluoride, etc.)
_____ Doctor Exam

Negotiable, if Time Permits

_____ Intra-oral Photos: For Treatment Presentation
_____ Diagnostic Impressions: Anterior/Cosmetic Restorations
_____ Fluoride
_____ Sealants
_____ Desensitizing Agent
_____ Anterior PAs

You can simplify and improve your Patient Experience by having clearly defined systems for each hygienist to follow.

We should have a patient task list for each hygiene patient. We see a real need to simplify the patient experience, and can do this by having clearly defined systems for each hygienist to follow.

In hygiene, it is amazing to me how few practices actually have a checklist of everything they want to happen every appointment. Flowcharts can help in many instances, especially with a new hire, but our flowcharts should evolve, and providers should have the flexibility and the freedom to do things out of order as long as everything gets done well.

Here is the Hygiene appointment flowchart we use:

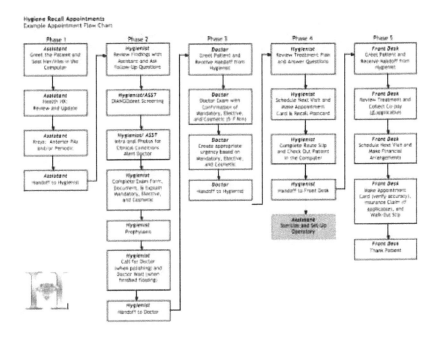

The flowchart is meant to be a guide. Some practices let the hygiene team accomplish these tasks in whatever order they deem most efficient but you will notice that there are both non-negotiable and negotiable standards. It is up to the dentists to determine what they consider non-negotiable standards, and communicate that to the team.

For the Preventative Therapist System, I might have non-negotiable standards of a risk assessment on each patient. (Actually this is the next key we will discuss in detail), fluoride acceptance above 80%, additional preventative therapies recommended based on risk, and following a consistent X-ray protocol. Those are what I personally would consider to be basic non-negotiable standards for a re-care appointment.

We should also have non-negotiable standards for the Periodontal Therapist Role. These might be a completed periodontal assessment on each patient, including probing a minimum of once per year, utilizing cutting-edge technology – like power-scalers and lasers.

It's not enough to just to treat Periodontal Disease; we also need to be measuring how well we're getting patients to accept it. So we should be tracking how well we are converting patients from proposed periodontal services to those that have actually completed those recommended services.

We also want to make sure that we're coding appropriately for services rendered. No alternating between periodontal maintenance and prophy visits, or other very common coding errors.

We must make sure that we are billing properly for the services we are doing.

Here are some examples of non-negotiable standards for the role of a Patient Treatment Advocate: use of the cavity-detecting lasers on every patient, every time. A virtual tour with an intra-oral camera and photos of at least three teeth shared with the patient. Restorative dentistry discussed utilizing tribal language (mandatory, elective, and cosmetic) and a World-Class transfer to the doctor.

These are just a few examples of the pieces of the systems that are needed to have sustainable success in hygiene.

Key #2: Begin with a Risk Assessment

For many in dentistry, we strive to do the very best for our patients. Our foundation is to serve our patients at the highest possible level, and when we focus on <u>how to serve </u>the patient at the highest possible level, production will follow.

If practices are struggling with patient acceptance of preventive services, we often find that they're not providing (or starting with) a risk assessment.

When we do the risk assessment correctly, all of a sudden the patient has very compelling and personal reasons why these services are of value. Our patients become engaged in the conversation but also in the solutions to help them improve their health.

It both motivates and inspires them to choose more services.

People often respond very well to photos. We use a lot of visual tools to help them understand what we see. Showing pictures with sugar cubes in the soda bottles to show how much sugar is in the beverages they're drinking, those are powerful.

Showing images with the PH threshold of waters and sodas and other drinks is also powerful.

Showing images of alkaline foods, a picture with celery and broccoli and peppers, and explaining how these foods can help naturally change the pH help us to gain patient engagement. Once they understand what to do differently and why they have had a struggle with cavities…we see things change. All of a sudden patients are willing to listen and move forward with preventive services.

Key #3: Tools

This is why the third key involved these images. We have created multiple tools that help with patient engagement in the treatment room. I have found that one of the most critical elements of patient education is helping them see WHY. WHY we have a problem and WHAT we can do about it. When people see things with their own eyes, they are more likely to believe. This is why using a set of chairside tools is important for each hygienist.

This toolkit could include:

- Risk Assessment Brochure… to download the brochure we use, go to: www.HygieneDiamonds.com/risk-assessment

- Periodontal Brochure

- Health Assessment worksheet

- A collection of laminated images that demonstrate and educate the patient about where they are and what we can do to prevent future problems.

The sugar in popular drinks:

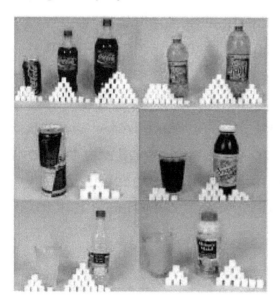

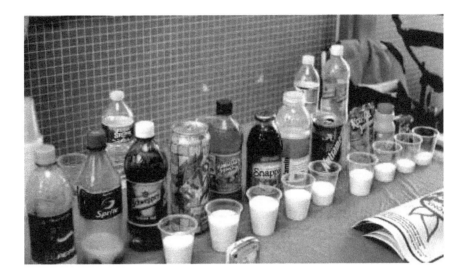

PH Levels:

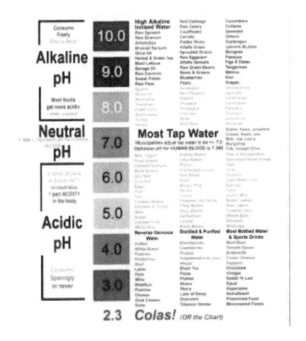

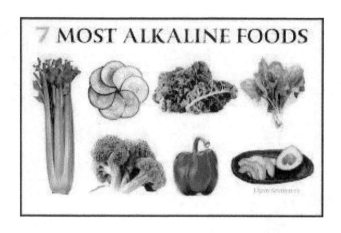

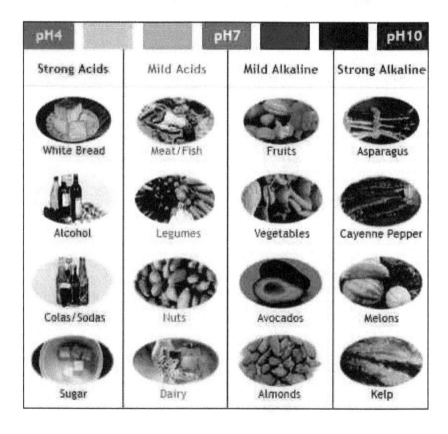

This is why, using a set of chair side tools is important for each hygienist. When we do this, we elevate effectiveness in patient understanding, compliance, and acceptance.

Key #4: Developing a Hygiene Leader

If you're not satisfied with the level of consistency of either productivity or tasks associated with the standard of care in your hygiene department, you should look to develop a hygiene leader.

If you only have one hygienist, then, of course, they're responsible personally for what's happening to hygiene. Once there are multiple providers, it's often helpful to have one go-to individual that is our leader for the hygiene team.

So what does your hygiene leader do?

First, we need to be able to clearly define what we think high performance looks like. What metrics are we looking for? What do we really want to see? Then we need to facilitate that performance and establish how to encourage that performance.

The hygiene team leader is someone who can step in and really help us manage and lead that department. They should plan, organize, direct and coordinate all the activities of the hygienists and Hygiene Assistants (if applicable) engaged in dental hygiene activities.

In addition, they can oversee the implementation of all critical systems, the completion of projects in hygiene, and high-performing important duties. With the right leadership structure, we can see tremendous growth. We have also seen limited growth and a struggle to perform well without good leadership.

I have found it works much better if the hygiene team leader is also a hygienist. I've seen chaos when we have someone who is not a hygienist trying to lead the hygiene team.

Here's what the hygiene team leader can do.... They serve as a member of the leadership management team. In conjunction with the president, the practice administrator, and other team leaders, they would participate in strategic and operational planning for the organization.

Based on the company's strategic and operational plans, the hygiene team leader would work on reporting with personnel to set goals and objective, as well as operational strategies.

They help the hygiene department achieve specific goals and objectives assigned to the hygiene team leader's area of responsibility.

They're responsible for managing the hygienists and hygiene assistants in an effort to bring your company's strategic and operational goals and objectives to fruition.

We want the hygiene team leader to be hyper focused on consistency. They are going to make sure that they're setting the methods and the work systems for a hygienist to improve productivity and determine reasons for production difficulties. When things don't go as planned, the Hygiene team leader will dive in and try to identify what's going on.

They can analyze cost and production records to ensure that their piece of the operation is efficient and profitable. They can ensure the implementation of policies, procedures, and practices required to provide quality patient care.

The hygiene team leader can also institute measures or approve suggestions to improve efficiency on operational working conditions. They are really the conduit between the hygienist in the trenches and the leadership of the practice.

Once you have multiple providers, this becomes a critical element to achieving sustainable success. It's having one go-to person who's really helping direct the hygiene team and develop the people in the trenches every day.

It doesn't mean that the hygiene team leader is not also in the trenches. We have practices who have their hygiene team leader still seeing patients three days a week but has half a day per week to handle their hygiene team leader responsibilities.

Once practices are developing it can be incredibly beneficial to manage and inspire world-class consistency in hygiene through developing a Hygiene Team Leader. If we expand beyond multiple providers and have multiple locations, we need a regional director of hygiene to oversee more than six locations.

So when we look at strategic growth and planning, leadership is a key element here and too often is overlooked when it comes to the hygiene department.

Key #5: Hygiene Compensation

This one is so important, we will go in depth about it in the next chapter.

Wendy Briggs

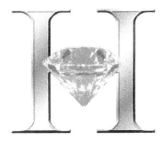

CHAPTER 9

HOW TO HIRE AND DEVELOP SUPER-STAR HYGIENISTS

Compensation Models for Hygiene

One of the most common questions I get is how to find and hire exceptional team members. I think the most common way to find them is to develop them!

There are certainly some things we have learned over the years about hiring and developing high-performing hygienists, and one of the most critical elements is compensation. This is often why hygienists don't achieve high levels of productivity consistently. We haven't made it worthwhile to do so.

It is critical that practices have some type of production-based compensation in place. Hourly pay can breed laziness in many employees but especially in producers.

Many doctors experience frustration with hygiene and hygiene productivity because their compensation structure has never been set up as a win-win.

Creating a Win-Win for Everyone

Many hygiene providers are wary of production-based compensation because there are many things outside of their control. It can be frightening having to depend completely on someone else to fill your schedule when it has a direct impact on your paycheck. Also, some practices try to compensate based on collections and find that is often unsustainable. Too many decisions that affect collections are outside the hygiene providers control. It can be demotivating over time.

The essential structure of an effective compensation model should have:

• A security net so they don't panic. Most hygienists are reluctant to go full commission even though that's how they can get the maximum amount of compensation in a well-run practice. There is not a safety net, and we often need that to feel comfortable.

• More compensation on higher production days. When hygienists work hard and do well with promoting same-day, preventive services or periodontal services, they know there's something in it for them at the end of the day. This creates a more productive employee from the beginning.

The Formula for hygienists without an Assistant:

Here's a simple transition formula that works best with hygienists who don't have an assistant.

The accepted principle is that hygienists should produce about three times what they earn. In recent years though, insurance adjustments have been growing. We find it might be necessary to pad the daily base if you participate with insurance. This enables you to be profitable,

- **The Daily Base.** Set the daily base at 3.5-4 times (depending on how many insurance write offs you have) what the hygienist is being paid.

- **Additional Compensation.** Anything they produce above that number, compensate them an additional 10% or 15%. This varies based on other incentives or benefits you have in place: If they're part of a team bonus, it may only be 10%; if this is their only incentive, offer a higher percentage. To illustrate, if they're currently making $300 a day, their daily base is $1050. When they produce above $1050, they receive the additional percentage. Their hourly salary stays the same, but if they are profitable, there's something extra in it for them at the end of that day.

The Formula for hygienists with an assistant:

If the hygienist has an assistant, adjust the formula in this way:

Add your hygienist's salary to your assistant's salary and multiply by 3.5-4. If they already average $1,500 a day with an assistant, it doesn't make sense to have the daily rate start at $1,000. So this is a guideline that you can utilize to make sure your daily base is not below what you need to be profitable.

Underlying Principles in the Formula

Decide on a base that makes sense from a financial standpoint but don't set the base too high.

Remember, you're not giving them 100% of what they produce above that base. It's only 10% or 15%. There's still plenty of profitability left for the practice, even after that additional percentage is paid. Every additional dollar of production, the overhead on that dollar decreases as you go.

If you set the base too high, it's demoralizing. The hygiene team will look at it and say, "We're never going to hit that."

This needs to be figured daily. Don't average out production over the month or the quarter. You lose the power of immediacy when you do that. This model has proven very effective.

In one large corporate organization, they had a complex bonus that was calculated over a long period of time. It was too complex and unmotivating. Before we shifted to a daily incentive, 26% of their hygienists were earning a bonus. After we switched to a daily formula, the very next month 100% of their hygienists had earned a bonus. It works.

Avoid the Knee-Jerk Reaction... Don't Nickel and Dime

"My hygienist is already making plenty of money. I don't want to pay them anymore" is a common knee-jerk reaction.

Sometimes we focus on the wrong number. When you actually run the numbers, even though you're writing out an additional amount to your hygienist, the practice is often much farther ahead than where it would have been if production had not increased. The more they take home, the more the doctor takes home.

The more production they provide, the more profit there is in the practice in general. It's incentive for the hygiene team to be productive. When they are more productive, everyone wins. Especially the patient, because to increase productivity, patient care has improved.

When practices go from an hourly wage to production-based compensation, the productivity, energy level, and happiness of employees jumps. That means more patients are being taken care of in a better way.

Even after implementation of the compensation model, some doctors still drag their feet.

Take the leap. Don't nickel and dime. Don't worry.

Production jumps significantly once these changes are made. It's often 30%–40% overnight. When you combine the compensation shift with the systems we teach, we see a literal explosion of hygiene productivity.

Production will increase dramatically if this was the only change you made and nothing else was implemented.

Attracting the Right Candidates

Be clear about what you're looking for. You want someone who has these traits:

- Patient-focused

- A team player

- Energetic and enthusiastic

- Thrive under an incentive program

- Good at talking to people

- A winning attitude

- Will flourish in a team environment

Hire for Personality: I believe you should hire for personality. You can teach the rest, of the, necessary skills. Look more for personality than the skill sets on the resume.

Detecting Personality: Personality is hard to detect just by looking at a resume or sometimes even on the phone.

Use a Temp Agency: We all have hygienists that need days off. Have temps come in and replace them when it's time to hire someone; find those people who filled in and did an excellent job—the ones who everyone liked and got along with.

Approach Your Staff: Often, team members have friends, associates, or school classmates who may be looking for a hygienist position. Personal recommendations from trusted people should carry a certain weight.

Use Careful Wording in Your Ads: The words you're using in the ad help weed out many potential applicants who may not fit what you're looking for.

Using words in the ad such as "highly motivated," "patient- focused," "team player," and so on are going to weed out those who just want the 9:00 to 5:00 paycheck. If you're not highly motivated, what are the odds you're going to respond to an ad that advertises "highly motivated?"

It's not a bad idea to mention in the ad or tell applicants initially that it's a production-based compensation structure. If they're not interested in functioning under that structure, chances are they're not highly motivated.

Mention your Delivery Method: "You're going to be working hand in hand with a highly trained assistant who'll make your job easier once you're providing services for our patients." Some hygienists may not want to use that delivery model.

That helps everyone to be very clear on what's expected.

Interview Questions for Providers: These questions determine the winning attitude and identify top hygienists.

- Ask what their production averages are. If

they know that number off the top of their head, it's a solid indicator of a good prospect. They're on top of what they personally can provide. Note: If they don't know their numbers, it doesn't mean they're not a good prospect. It's either positive or neutral.

- Ask about their familiarity with current techniques. Are they trained and have they used a laser (if it is permissible in your state)? Are they familiar with the software you're using? And so on. These are going to help you know how much training needs to happen.

- Ask about their continuing education in recent years and who it was with. This shows the philosophies they've been trained with, and it helps you ascertain their personality as well.

- Ask why they left their last office or are looking for new work. This can give you a glimpse into their personality and help you avoid some trouble down the road.

- Ask what they have done in their past and what they are willing to do for you in the future.

- "Are you willing to give injections on behalf of the doctor?" (assuming that it's legal in your state)

- "Are you comfortable taking impressions?"

- "How long has it been since you placed a sealant? Are you comfortable placing sealants?" We've worked with hygienists who haven't placed a sealant in 20 years. Can they learn how to do it again? Are they willing to? Some are. Some aren't.

- "Are you willing to donate your time toward charitable efforts?"

- "Are you willing to donate your time to a 'Dentistry with a Heart' event?"

Are They Demanding or Accommodating? Do they make demands or do they ask what you want?

Sometimes, a hygienist will come in and say, "If I'm going to work here, I have to have this and this." That's an indicator that you may not have the right fit.

The "Whatever It Takes" Exercise

This seems random, but it is a tried-and-true tactic.

On the way to the interview location, whether it's in the doctor's office or wherever it may be, have a trash can in view. Have a piece of paper crumpled up in a ball on the floor next to the trash can.

If the person stops, picks it up and throws it away, it tells you a lot about their personality, that:

- They're willing to do whatever it takes.

- They take the initiative to fix a problem when they see one.

- They don't have to be asked.

- They're motivated.

- They pay attention to detail.

There's a lot you can tell from that simple exercise.

Team Member Involvement: Many times the doctor is the only one involved in the hiring process, but the opinions of your team matter, especially with a provider.

During the hiring process, include other hygienists in the practice and the hygiene assistants they're going to be working with directly. They often have a better insight into the team player quality than you will. They get a feel for the person much faster than a doctor will.

Applicants usually show the doctor a little different side of themselves than they show the staff; it's just a part of human nature. By involving your team, you'll get more knowledge because your team will see things you're blind to.

Working Interviews:

With many employees, a working interview isn't a good idea. With a hygienist, it's almost critical to have one.

When it comes to a provider, you need to have at least a few days where you can test them out and they can test you out before there's an offer or a permanent contract.

You don't have to call it a working interview. You can pay them temporary wages, but they need to come in and work a couple of days.

There are things you can't tell from their resume or

the job interview. For example, you need to see how timely they are and how well they work with your team members.

See How Hygienists are with Patients

You need to see how they are with patients—how they talk to patients, how they treat patients, and how patients respond to them.

Patient feedback should be a critical component of the hiring process. Take surveys of the patients after they're finished.

It's even a wise strategy to have a couple of ringers as their patients. Ringers are people who will be brutally honest with you about their treatment. They need to tell you if it was painful. Did they like the hygienist? Were they friendly and warm?

A hygienist often has your patient's undivided attention for 30 to 60 minutes. Having a hygiene provider that's not a good fit can cause some damage to the practice. If you've got someone who's causing your patients a lot of discomfort or pain, patients will start leaving in droves.

Hygienists Need to See if it is the Right Fit for Them

They'll see if your delivery model suits them. It may not.

The hygienist may want an assisted model, for example. If they expect an assistant to help them to type data, it's something you both need to know from the beginning.

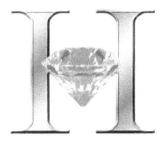

Chapter 10

Why it Hasn't Worked in the Past

Many doctors have tried to make changes in their hygiene departments only to encounter resistance and since none of us like confrontation, they give up. You've probably felt this when trying to implement new things in the office – not just in hygiene.

But let's take a look at it from your team's perspective.... It could be that you had consultants work with them who really don't understand hygiene. Maybe you came back, all excited, from a seminar and announced, "This is what we need to do differently,"

But there was never a clear pathway showing HOW to get that done. I can't tell you how many times I've heard from doctors who say, "I've asked my hygienist to do this for years, and it just doesn't happen."

When I am able to sit down with the hygiene team and explain the compelling reasons why the change should happen and I have backed that up with science, with the position of the ADA and the ADHA it gives them a reason to change. We have a discussion about why this makes sense, and then show them HOW to do it.

It's amazing what happens to their willingness to accept new ideas. I would also say that many hygienists are more than willing, but no one has shown them HOW to get these things done.

But My Hygienist Won't Listen to Me

Here's the thing. If you really want to see and inspire change in hygiene, you need to be the true leaders of this change.

It's not enough just to pass off the books to the hygiene team or to send them to a course or seminar without you.

You need to be on the same page as your team – this means that you need to hear the same ideas, concepts, changes in our profession.

You need to be leading the change

You can't have people all rowing a boat going different directions. In order to really make progress, we all have to be rowing in the same direction; we have to be rowing together; we have to be working together. Too often dentists treat hygiene as a separate entity within their practice, and it really shouldn't be that way.

Hygiene can drive the growth of the rest of the practice, if both the dentist and the hygienists are in alignment on where the practice is going and how you're going to get there. As the leader and the CEO of the practice, you need to be involved in the discussions so that you can support the initiatives that hygiene is trying to accomplish. Once you have determined the goals, this is the point in which you can step aside and let your team drive the new initiatives, but asking them to drive before you have indicated where they should go is the recipe for failure.

So How Do You Do It?

Well, for starters, whenever you participate in a training course, it should be both the hygienists and the dentists together. Then I would start with setting goals together.

One of the most powerful things I do as a consultant is to open the lines of communication. I like to start by setting a standard of care for your practice. This opens the doorway and leads the discussions for the dentist and the hygienist to get on the same page. Once the hygienists know the vision of the doctor, they feel more secure and less likely to be resistant to change and are happy to do what's necessary to get there.

What is often lacking is no one in the practice -- hygienist or other team members -- know where the doctor is going. Setting goals in hygiene are as easy as having a conversation with the hygiene team about "This is where we'd like to go," and "This is my ideal. This is how the ideal patient experience should go," or "This is what I think our non-negotiable standards of care should be."

Once the goals are set and the lines of communication have been opened, you need to add a measure of accountability. Goals without metrics are just wishes.

The accountability starts with the morning huddle and continues through team meetings. We are checking every day our progress on the goals that we've set. We're celebrating accomplishments and saying thank you. Giving high fives when we do accomplish a goal, that is the fun part!

It's amazing how far a "thank you," a high-five, even a quick note at the end of the day will go. Everyone likes a little recognition for a job well done.

The Difference Between Leading
and Micro Managing

Being involved and being a leader are very different. People don't want to be managed; they want to be led. I've seen doctors that are really good at leading their hygiene team, celebrating the accomplishments

I would suggest that micro-managing your providers is an incredibly costly approach. An example of this would be highlighting every missed piece of calculus. A good leader will watch to see if this becomes a trend and will then create a discussion using the standards of care as their basis to make a correction.

Conversations should happen away from the treatment room. That conversation then goes something like this … "I'm concerned. I'm seeing some areas of calculus that have been missed. What do you think we should do about this?" "What can we do to help support you so that you feel like you have the time you need to remove deposits?" That's the conversation that a leader would have.

You never want to handle a situation like this in front of the patient. Highlighting a mistake or a misstep in front of a patient is a symptom of a micro-manager. Instead of catching your people doing something wrong, we should be focused on catching them doing something right! This pays off huge in the long run.

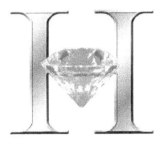

CHAPTER 11

"Dentists are Just Greedy"…

I am a moderator on some online hygiene forums. It seems like almost every day, there are hygienists on the forum posting about how frustrating practicing dental hygiene is in today's world.

They are often of the opinion that dentists are greedy and it's all about the money.

I believe that this opinion comes from years of miscommunication and misunderstanding of the Business of Dentistry and more importantly the Business of Dental Hygiene.

Let's first talk about the misunderstanding of the Business of Dentistry and Dental Hygiene...

I've always believed that if we take care of the patient at the highest possible level and give patients the opportunity to choose more for themselves, then the production will naturally follow.

There's really no need to focus on the money or the production if we're doing the best possible thing for the patients. However, money is the only metric that we have to measure how well we are providing for our patients.

I often hear hygienists saying, "*We're in health care. We shouldn't have to worry about money.*" In a perfect world, nobody would ever have to worry about money, but that's not reality.

The reality is every dental office has overhead and a cost to serving patients. Every practice has bills to pay. Every dentist needs to pay the hygienist's salary. If we aren't focused on the production at least a little bit, then we stand a chance of going out of business.

In just 2009 alone, more than 600 dentists went bankrupt or closed their doors in Phoenix, Arizona. More dentists went bankrupt in 2009 than in any year since the Great Depression. It wasn't limited to the recession; it still happens every day.

Your hygienists, and your entire team for that matter, need to recognize that production matters and being efficient matters. If the practice succeeds, then everyone wins. The patient wins, the team members win, the hygienists win, and the doctors win.

I think that the key here is finding balance. Finding a balance between patient care, patient service, serving our patients to the highest possible level, and realizing that when we do that, the production does take care of itself.

We all entered dentistry as a profession because we wanted to help people and serve people. The key is just finding the balance so that everybody feels we are doing the right thing.

Some consultants and experts may not have what is best for the patient as the most important element.

Sadly, many have never practiced dentistry and aren't responsible personally for patient health. They have never grown a practice, provided hygiene services, and really don't know what it takes. I have heard some really bad advice, and sadly sometimes we follow that bad advice with disastrous results.

What I am trying to say is that most dentists I have talked to and worked with are NOT greedy. They may be guilty of listening to bad advice, but rarely do I see someone who is willing to sacrifice patient care for the money.

Let's talk about the misunderstandings that cause this...

The book Men are from Mars, Women are from Venus was written to bridge the gap in communication and understanding between men and women. No one has written a book to bridge the gap between dentists and hygienists and team members.

As a successful dentist and business owner, you are always seeking out the new ways to do everything in the practice from learning the newest insurance codes, to training on the newest lasers, to the newest practice management strategies, to the newest hygiene tools. Your goal is to grow your business and provide your team with the best tools to accomplish their jobs.

Imagine this very common scenario:

Often (with good intentions) dentists come back from training or from the webinar you just listened to and announce ….

"Our hygienists need to be producing 30% of practice production," or

"We need to be doing sealants on all adults," or

"Our periodontal average should be around 20%,"

When asked why they should be doing that they hear, "The speaker said we should." Then they say that insurance won't pay for it.

What they really heard was "Because we (and by "we" I mean the doctor) want to make more money."

Not only do we have a misunderstanding to the WHY we are doing things, most times there has been no training or understanding as to HOW we are going to do it. Knowing what we should do and truly mastering it are two different things.

For every new service that a practice implements, we have seen the need to have scripts created and training to help the team understand the WHY. Why are you now offering this service (why didn't you offer this in the past) and how will this affect the patient? When teams understand the WHY and are given the HOW they become unstoppable.

Communication and miscommunication isn't just limited to inside the practice. The key to increasing productivity in hygiene is often just in communicating with the patients at a higher level, **why** they need what we are recommending and **what** benefits they stand to see in that. When we start communicating like this, the turnaround is immediate.

It's incredibly powerful, what we can do with just one day in many practices. When we start focusing on higher-level services and when the practices commit to learning and implementing these over time, that's when we start to see true mastery.

Understanding the Business of Dental Hygiene has helped countless practices realize levels of productivity and patient care they never thought possible.

This is the most fulfilling element to what I do. Helping dentists and hygienists know what to do to uncover the hidden diamonds beneath their feet is rewarding. "Success isn't just about what you accomplish in your life, it's about what you inspire others to do." -unknown

.

ABOUT THE AUTHOR

Wendy Briggs has been called the *"World's most famous hygienist."* She is a practicing hygienist, strategic advisor, speaker, trainer, consultant, and coach. She has directly influenced more than 3,718 dental practices in 12 countries around the world. She has the longest proven track record of helping dentists and hygienists double hygiene production.

She has consulted and worked with some of the biggest and fastest growing private dental practices, as well as some of the largest DSO organizations in both the United States and Australia, including Heartland Dental, Breakaway Practice, Mortenson Dental, & Dental Corp. She is the recommended hygiene consultant for Henry Schein Dental.

As a speaker she has shared the stage with every 'name' in dentistry including; Dr. Tom Orent, Woody Oakes, Scott Leune of Breakaway Practice, and The Dawson Academy. She has presented at the Chicago Midwinter Meeting, the Yankee Dental Meeting, the Greater New York Dental Meeting, the Townie Meeting, Rocky Mountain Dental Implant Institute, the Big Apple Meeting, CDA in San Francisco, the Laser Clinicians meeting, and the Academy for General Dentists.

Hygiene is her passion... and exploding hygiene productivity and profits are her areas of expertise.

Next Steps:

Hygiene is no longer just about saving teeth, but saving lives, and you are no longer just a dentist but a *physician of the mouth.* Among our clients, we are producing numbers in hygiene that are breaking records, yet our hygienists have more energy at the end of the day and feel more satisfied with the service they provide than they ever have in the past.

We have scoured over hundreds, even thousands of practice analysis reports from practices in small towns, like Denham Springs, LA to downtown Manhattan, and in each practice we have found a minimum of $150,000 of lost opportunity. But more important to us, the lost opportunity to provide your patients with the level of care that they deserve. Each report is like an MRI of the practice; within minutes we can see what's happening and quickly diagnose the problem and provide solutions.

The biggest challenge that you face in creating a hygiene-driven practice will be getting your hygienists on board with the changes. Let me come alongside you and your hygiene team to show you what's possible.

The first step is to schedule your Hygiene Productivity Assessment. During this call, we will complete a comprehensive analysis of your current practice and personalize a plan for you to double your current hygiene production.

Get started by requesting your Hygiene Productivity Assessment at www.HygieneProductivityAssessment.com